SAFETY

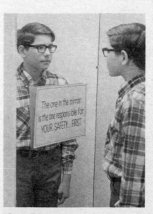

1976 Printing of the
1971 Revision

**BOY SCOUTS OF AMERICA
NORTH BRUNSWICK, NEW JERSEY**

Requirements

1. Prepare a safety notebook. Include:

   a. Newspaper and other stories showing main kinds of accidents.

   b. Similar materials showing five causes of accidents.

   c. The approximate yearly loss for main kinds of accidents in terms of deaths, injuries, and cost in dollars.

   d. How a serious fire or accident involving you or your parents can change your life.

   e. How safe practices and safety devices make your life easier and more pleasurable.

2. At three appropriate and safe locations spend 3 hours observing and listing safe and unsafe practices by (a) motor vehicle drivers, (b) pedestrians, (c) bicycle riders, (d) passengers (car, bus, train, or plane). Show this list to your counselor.

3. Do the following:

   a. Using a safety checklist approved by your counselor, make an inspection of your home. Explain the hazards found, why they are hazards, and how they can be corrected.

   b. Review your family's plan of escape in case of fire in your home.

4. Sketch your troop meeting place (or another public building where people gather) and show exits. Are they adequate? Show which exit you would use in an emergency. Explain what should be done in a panic.

Copyright © 1971
Boy Scouts of America
North Brunswick, New Jersey
Library of Congress Catalog Card Number: 19-600
ISBN 0-8395-3347-0
No. 3347   Printed in U.S.A.   30M376

5. Make two safety checklists, one each for school and recreation. Include 10 points on each.

6. Make a plan for an accident prevention program for the following outdoor situations: (a) camping and hiking, (b) storm and wind, (c) water activities. Each plan should include an analysis of possible hazards, proposed action to correct the hazards, and reasons for the correction you propose.

7. Do one of the following:

   a. Report on a safety project that you helped to plan or took part in.

   b. Go with a company representative on a safety inspection tour of his company's premises (plant or other place where people work). Make a report.

   c. Join a building or fire inspector on an inspection tour of a public building. Make a report.

   d. Plan a farm safety project to correct unsafe conditions and equipment hazards.

8. Tell how you contribute to the safety of yourself, your family, and your community.

Contents

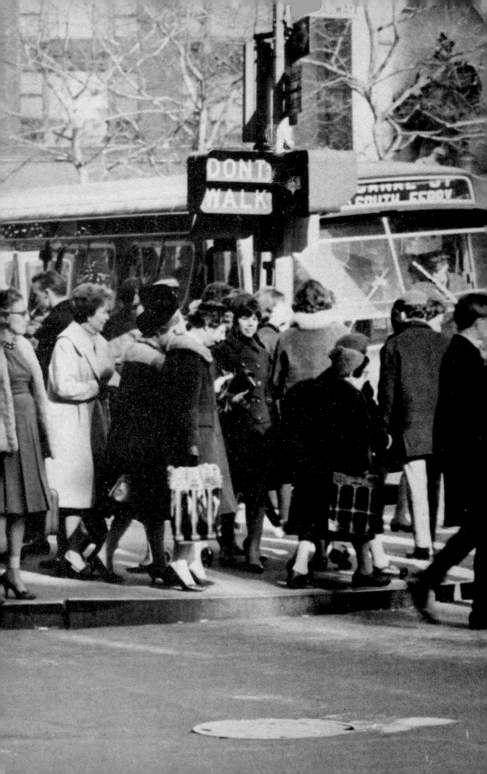

Safety Is a Way of Life

1. Prepare a safety notebook. Include:

   a. Newspaper and other stories showing main kinds of accidents.

   b. Similar materials showing five causes of accidents.

   c. The approximate yearly loss for main kinds of accidents in terms of deaths, injuries, and cost in dollars.

   d. How a serious fire or accident involving you or your parents can change your life.

   e. How safe practices and safety devices make your life easier and more pleasurable.

Safety, like Scouting, is a way of life. It demands a set of goals. Sure, staying alive and well and keeping yourself and your things in one piece are important, but doing things safely means that you will finish what you started out to do and get some pleasure out of doing it.

You can think of safety in two ways: what it means to you and what it means to others.

Think of your own personal safety. If you can avoid accidents, you can finish what you start. You can do the things you want to do.

A boy liked swimming more than anything else he did, but he also liked to walk barefoot. Early one summer he cut his foot on a broken bottle in the road. No swimming all summer! One accident took away his greatest pleasure. Do you think it had to happen?

Another boy allowed an accident to hurt him even more. Riding his bike carelessly after dark with no lights, he was struck by a car. After months in the hospital and at home, he was back to normal—almost. But he can never take part in sports again. He has a leg injury that can't be corrected.

So safety is in your own interest. If you keep yourself safe, you can do the things you enjoy. As a Scout, you also have a duty to other people. Accidents happen to them, too, and you can help prevent them.

Someone smashes a glass jar in the road. You sweep

it up. A child might have cut himself. A car's tire might have been cut and blown out later. A simple act on your part made somebody safer.

You go swimming at a public beach. You see a small child swimming too far from shore. You go out and swim with him to a safer depth. You're not a hero— or are you?

Safety involves you and other people.

What Causes Accidents

People sometimes think that accidents just happen. They're just bad luck or they come out of nowhere. If one happens to you, that's the breaks. Don't you believe it.

An accident is not intended to happen. It is not planned. It is not deliberate. But that doesn't mean that an accident has no cause. Every accident is caused.

An accident can be caused by an unsafe condition. Bad brakes on a car or an icy sidewalk are unsafe conditions by which an accident is more likely to happen.

An accident can also be caused by unsafe acts. These are not "conditions." They're what someone does or fails to do. If you jump off the roof of a house or ride your bike through a red light, you are doing an unsafe act.

An unsafe condition, all by itself, can cause an accident. An unsafe act, alone, can also cause an accident. Do you think an accident could be caused by both an unsafe act and an unsafe condition? Of course.

Suppose you have weak brakes on your bike. That's an unsafe condition. You ride fast up to an intersection and put on your brakes too late. That's an unsafe act. The bike doesn't stop, and you run into a moving car.

Wherever you are there may be unsafe conditions. Whoever you are sometimes you may be guilty of unsafe acts.

What causes people to act unsafely? It's easy to say "carelessness," but that's not saying much. Here are some of the real reasons:
• taking chances—fooling around ("I'll slip by just this once.")
• being unprepared ("I didn't think we'd need a map.")
• fatigue ("The late show was good, but I'm sure tired today.")

6

- overconfidence ("Of course I can swim a mile.")
- haste ("If I hadn't been running, I wouldn't have slipped.")
- fear ("I couldn't move.")
- excitement ("Hurry up and light it.")
- the lure of the forbidden ("No Swimming Here")
- not knowing the rules ("You mean I shouldn't have stood up in the canoe?")
- ignoring the rules ("I didn't know it was loaded.")

The above reasons are some of the "mental" causes of unsafe acts. But some people often do things unsafely because they are "not themselves" or are not in good condition. How do they get that way? Here are some reasons:
- drug abuse (including misuse of doctors' prescriptions)
- alcohol
- poor hearing or vision
- illness
- temporary handicaps such as broken limbs

Safety Means Knowing How

Safety does not necessarily mean a total absence of accidents. Risks are everywhere. People are killed just crossing the street. But risks are voluntary actions and can be managed. Emergencies can be met and handled, but it takes know-how. What you can't prevent, you usually can compensate for or protect against.

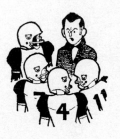

That is what safety does, but what is it? Safety is doing whatever you want or need to do and doing it right. It is playing football the way it is supposed to be played and enjoying it. Football coaches tell us that the one who gets injured is the one who does not play the game energetically or the one who does not wear the right protective equipment. Safety is the skill, the practiced knowledge, that makes almost anything possible. It is not worrying about deep water when you know how to swim and can handle the distance—but it is being aware of undertow and always having a buddy. Safety is seeing and overcoming hazards.

Facts About Accidents

Safety experts classify accidents into four categories: motor vehicle, work, home, and public. The public category excludes motor vehicle and work accidents in public places, includes sports and recreation (swimming, hunting, etc.), air, water, or land transportation except motor vehicle, and public building accidents.

According to the National Safety Council, in one recent year accidents killed 116,000 and injured 10,-800,000 Americans. This is more than the deaths of U.S. military personnel in the Korean War and the Vietnam War combined. The dollar cost was high too —over $23 billion!

Here is how the accidents in that year were divided up.* Some deaths and injuries are included in more than one classification. (The U.S. population that year was about 200 million people.)

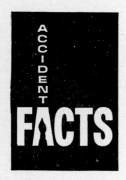

	*Killed	*Injured
Motor vehicle	56 thousand	2 million
Work	14 thousand	2.2 million
Home	27 thousand	4 million
Public	21 thousand	2.7 million

Here's another way of looking at the same figures:
• One person in 20 was injured or killed in an accident.
• One person in every 100 was injured or killed by a motor vehicle.
• People are twice as safe at work than they are at home.

How safe are boys your age? In an average year over 2,800 boys ages 10 to 14 die in accidents in the United States. Such deaths happen in these proportions:

Type	Percent
Motor vehicle	42.1
Drowning	21.0
Firearms	10.8
Fires and explosions	4.0
Falls	2.1
All other	20.0

NOTE: For additional facts about accidents, try these sources:
Encyclopaedia Britanica or *World Book*
National Safety Council publications
Local, county, or state health departments

What Accidents Can Do to You

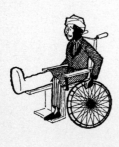

It's not hard to imagine adding yourself to the accident statistics. Any day's newspaper tells at least one tragic story of someone's accident. In every case the victim was somebody who didn't plan or expect to be hurt or killed.

In a matter of seconds everything you were ever going to do and be can be snuffed out. At the very least you suffer pain and inconvenience from an accident.

At worst, an accident kills or damages you for life.

Safety saves you, but it does more than that. Mix each safety ingredient with some of the things you like to do, such as swim, play ball, or hike, and you will see they really cook up honest-to-goodness pleasure.

One ingredient is knowledge and skill. Who enjoys swimming more: the fellow who knows how to or the one who never bothered to learn and is afraid to wade more than 2 feet from shore? Perhaps a lifesaving device would help. Who plays the game better and with more pleasure: the boy who knows what he is doing or the joker who is floundering around? And who knows the real thrill of the trails and the mountains and profits more while worrying less: the one who has the safety know-how or the one who is backing a hunch?

A second ingredient is the inquiring mind that looks ahead. A person who is out on a raft and is aware that a storm is coming and the one who is not: Who has the easier—and safer—swim to shore? A person doing a job who uses the right tools and one who does not: Who has the simpler, more pleasant job ahead? Who has the more pleasant and safe time: the one who plans his trip, checks for weather conditions, and goes prepared or the one who does not?

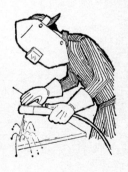

A third ingredient is knowing and accepting your limitations. Two equal swimmers eye a distant objective. One knows he can reach it but that it will be a long haul. The other decides the girl on the distant shore is worth it, but is not sure that he can make it. He either walks 3 miles and decides to be "safe" and lose the girl, or, over-confident, he plunges ahead, only to find fear and possible panic as, halfway there, too late to turn back, he begins to wonder whether he can reach the shore or not.

A boy taking manual arts, unaware of his limitations, ignores safety guards or a holder for drilling that small piece of metal or wood. He risks losing his fingers and winds up with a rejected piece of work. But the fellow next to him knows that for fine work he needs the holder and for his own safety he needs the guard as well as safety goggles. Using them he zips through a perfect piece—without an accident, without a rejection.

On a hike or camping trip there are two very different Scouts: the Scout who just picks up his pack without checking its contents or anything else and the Scout who plans and prepares.

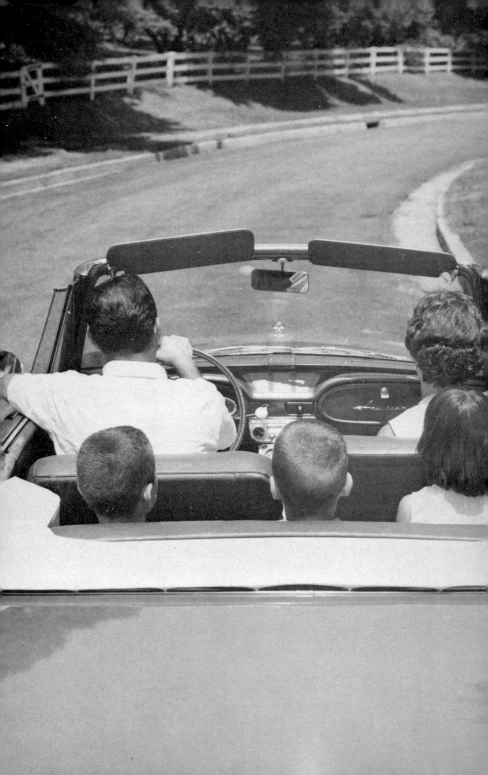

Safety on the Move

2. At three appropriate and safe locations spend 3 hours observing and listing safe and unsafe practices by (a) motor vehicle drivers, (b) pedestrians, (c) bicycle riders, (d) passengers (car, bus, train, or plane). Show this list to your counselor.

Appropriate and Safe Locations

An appropriate location is one that will enable you to observe what you're there to see. A dead-end street would not be appropriate, but a superhighway might be. A safe location is one where you won't be in danger yourself. (You could see a lot from the white line in the middle of a busy highway, but it's not a safe place to spend 3 hours—or 3 minutes.)

A downtown street or a superhighway overpass would be good places to see motor vehicles. Downtown business streets are also good places to observe pedestrians and passengers. You know best where to see bicycle traffic.

Wherever you observe traffic, you will probably see more than one kind of vehicle. So you may want to make columns on your note pad or use a different page for motor vehicles, bikes, etc.

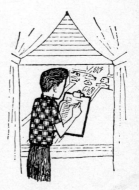

Remember that you are looking for both safe and unsafe acts. You'll have to keep them separate too. You may see a cyclist give a hand signal. That goes under bicycles, safe acts. You may see a motorist drive through a red light. That goes under motor vehicles, unsafe acts.

Where can you see best? For watching vehicles you may be able to see best from above. Perhaps you could observe downtown traffic from a stairway landing where a window gives you a good view of an intersection.

If there is a superhighway near your home, you might watch traffic from one of the bridges over it—providing there is a pedestrian walk.

Whatever observation posts you pick, be sure that they're safe for you. You certainly don't want to have an accident while working on the Safety merit badge!

Consider this possibility too. You could observe traffic while riding in a car. This would give you a chance to observe safe and unsafe acts of the driver as well as other drivers, pedestrians, and cyclists. But don't pick the worst driver you know to ride with. That wouldn't be a safe observation post.

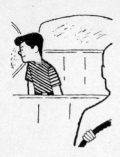

Vehicle Safety

This pamphlet cannot give you a full treatment of vehicle safety, because what is known would fill many books. Your best sources of information about driver safety are the *Automotive Safety* merit badge pamphlet and your state's traffic rule book (or driver's manual).

There are a good many wrong ideas about vehicle accidents. For example, we usually think of such accidents as two vehicles colliding. But a very large number of accidents involve only one vehicle. Sometimes that one vehicle is the only one around at the time of the accident. Another example: We think of the two vehicles colliding head-on or sideways at an intersection, but many collisions occur between two vehicles going in the same direction.

Still another wrong idea: Driving skill is being good at manipulating the car. Well, in part, it is; but the car travels in traffic and the rest of the driving skill involves driving safely in traffic. Being good at working the controls is just a part of driving skill.

Let's look at some typical traffic situations so you can see the kinds of judgment involved.

In figure 1 the driver of car B should allow 1 car length for each 10 miles of speed, or 5 car lengths if he is traveling at 50 miles per hour. Instead, he follows A at 2 car lengths. If A has to stop or slow suddenly, B will ram into A or run off the road or into the opposing lane.

In figure 2 there is a typical situation at an entrance to a superhighway. Car A is traveling normally at a reasonable speed. Car B is passing car A. So far, no problems. But car C is going to enter the right lane from the acceleration strip. In seconds, he will run out of pavement unless he swings left. If he does, he will hit car A in the side.

To play it safe, what should A, B, and C each do? Here are our suggestions. See if they're the same as yours.

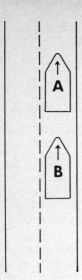

Figure 1

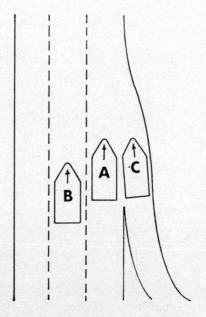

Figure 2

13

- A should accelerate, to leave space behind for C to enter.
- B should see what might happen and change to the far left lane after signaling.
- C should slow down, since he's the one who is going to run out of pavement if he doesn't.

Let's do one more. Look at figure 3.

The driver of car A knows the intersection and knows he has the right of way. He can see car B approaching. Being a skillful driver, the motorist in car A will (choose the correct decision):

- speed up and beat B to the intersection.
- assume B will stop and take no special precautions.
- take his foot off the accelerator and be ready to brake if B doesn't stop.
- stop at the intersection and wave B through.

While it's perfectly true that A has the right of way, there's no guarantee that B will stop. A cannot safely assume that. Being skillful, he knows enough not to speed through an intersection. It's safe to stop and wave B through, so A will be prepared to brake if B fails to stop.

As you observe motor vehicles, you will see very little evidence of great skill in manipulating the controls—mainly because not much is needed. But you will be able to see many examples of skill, or lack of it, in traffic situations like those illustrated. Here are some good examples of things to watch for:

GOOD	BAD
Smooth, even driving—no jerks or surprises	Fast starts and stops, abrupt changes of lane, weaving in and out
Allowing plenty of space	Driving too close to other vehicles
Signaling turns, stops, lane changes	Making changes without signaling
Slowing down in time	Last-minute panic stops
Obeying traffic rules and laws	Breaking rules and laws

Make a good, understandable list of the safe and unsafe driving acts you observe. Be ready to discuss the things on your list with your counselor.

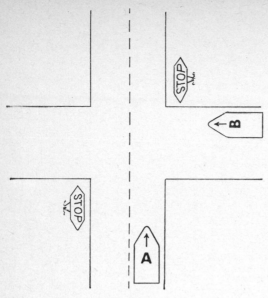

Figure 3

Pedestrian Safety

Walking is a skill people learn as babies. Yet there must be more to it than putting one foot ahead of the other. In one recent year 10 thousand American pedestrians were killed by motor vehicles. Pedestrians are about one-sixth of those killed by motor vehicles.

As you watch pedestrians from your observation posts, see how well they stick by these old reliable rules: (See figure 4, pages 16 and 17.)

- Cross streets only at intersections.
- Don't play in the street.
- At intersections with traffic lights, cross only at the green.
- Look for cars both ways and around the corner.
- Cross streets quickly, but don't run.
- Don't block your view with what you're carrying.
- At night, carry a light or something white.
- Walk on the left, facing traffic, if there are no sidewalks or curbs.
- Don't argue with the power, weight, and speed of a vehicle—even if you think you're right.

Following simple rules like these is the skill of being a pedestrian. In some communities the police make it

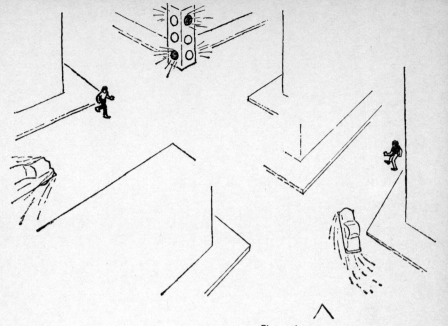

Figure 4

How many unsafe pedestrian a

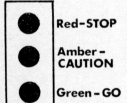

Red-STOP

Amber-CAUTION

Green-GO

easy to follow the rules by enforcing the laws affecting pedestrians very strictly. In some communities you would wait all day to see someone jaywalk or cross against a traffic light. In others, where enforcement is less strict, you may count hundreds of unsafe pedestrian acts in an hour.

Safety on a Bicycle

About 800 persons lose their lives and almost 150,000 others suffer disabling injuries in pedal cycling accidents in the United States each year. Yet collisions with motor vehicles account for only about 12 percent of all reported bicycle accidents. Also, it appears that there are a lot of ways of getting hurt on a bicycle. It also appears that ability to handle the bike has a lot to do with one's safety.

A bicycle can be a very dangerous vehicle. It can travel at respectable speeds and it offers no protection to the rider. It is no match for any motor vehicle in a collision. Who gets hurt, and where, and why?

Most bike accidents happen to children. That's be-

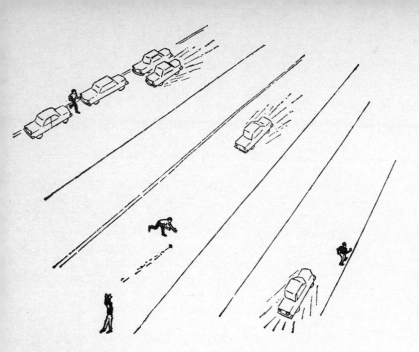

hown in these illustrations?

cause most bike riders are children. Five hundred of the 800 deaths noted above were children ages 5 to 14.

Where do bicycle accidents happen? The results of a study by the National Safety Council are shown in figure 5.

Between Intersections

About a third of bike accidents happen on a street between intersections. Relatively few of these involve a vehicle hitting a bike. Accidents in these locations seem to be caused mainly by what the cyclist does.

At Intersections

Many of these accidents happen to boys and girls ages 12, 13, and 14. Many more boys are involved than girls. Most happen between midafternoon and early evening.

On Driveways and Sidewalks

More girls than boys have bicycle accidents in driveways and on sidewalks. Younger riders have more accidents than older ones.

When you observe bicycle traffic, see if you can answer these questions:

• Why do cyclists run into vehicles between intersections?

• Why do so many interesection accidents happen to 12-, 13-, and 14-year-old cyclists?

• Why are more boys than girls injured at intersections?

• Why are more girls than boys injured in driveways and on sidewalks?

Another good guide for your observation, as well as your own safety, is the Scout Bicycle Safety Code.

Scout Bicycle Safety Code

• Follow local bicycle and traffic rules, signs, and lights.

• Keep to the right and ride in a straight line.

• Have a white light in front and a red light or reflector in back.

• Have a working signaling device such as a horn or a bell.

• Give pedestrians and automobiles the right-of-way. Avoid sidewalk riding.

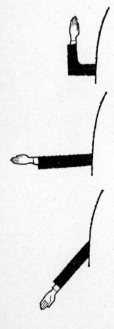

• Look out for parked cars pulling into traffic. Watch for pedestrians stepping out from parked cars. (The other guy can cause an accident too—unless you anticipate and are prepared for his mistakes.)

• Never hitch onto other vehicles. Never start or race in traffic.

• Carry no passenger. Do not carry objects that interfere with vision or control. Use a basket or bag for carrying school books.

• Make sure brakes are functioning smoothly. Keep bike in perfect operating condition.

• Slow down, look left and right at intersections.

• Always use proper hand signals for turning or stopping. (While accepted hand signals may vary from state to state, the most common are left turn—hand and arm extended horizontally; right turn—hand and arm extended upward; stop or decrease speed—hand and arm extended downward.

• Do not weave in and out of traffic or swerve from side to side.

• Dismount and walk bicycle across heavy traffic.

• Keep both hands on the handlebars except when signaling or shifting gears.

• Do not ride when you feel tired or ill.

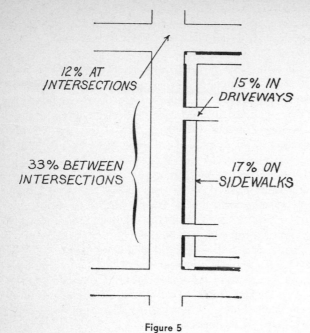

12% AT INTERSECTIONS

15% IN DRIVEWAYS

33% BETWEEN INTERSECTIONS

17% ON SIDEWALKS

Figure 5

Safety on Motorcycles, Scooters, Motorbikes, and Minibikes

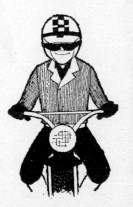

In most states, two-wheeled vehicles driven by a motor are treated by the law like automobiles. That is, the same rules apply as to insurance, licensed driver, and so forth. However, such vehicles can be and are ridden off public roads where traffic laws do not apply. It is not uncommon for young people to have serious accidents while operating them. For this reason this pamphlet contains information on such vehicles, even though most Scouts are too young to ride them on public roads.

Safety facts about motorcycles are true of the smaller vehicles even though their speed is less. Motor-driven bikes have two basic hazards. First, they have a lot of power in relation to their weight. Second, the rider is outside the vehicle and has no built-in protection.

An article in *Today's Health* magazine tells very well just what these hazards mean:

"The fact is, you can drive your car directly into another vehicle at, say, 10 miles an hour and, especially if your seat belt is fastened snugly, you most likely will not get hurt. Most adults have had this experience and they sometimes even joke about such minor mishaps.

"Now, in your imagination, place yourself upon the seat of a motorcycle and drive into traffic. An automobile makes a quick left turn in front of you and you put on your brakes, but you're still traveling about 10 miles an hour when you impact the side of the car. Now it's a different story—instead of receiving a jolting thump and a tug of a seat belt, then settling back into soft upholstery, you're catapulted high into the air, literally flying right over the car your cycle hit. And, if you don't smash right into a lamp pole, a street sign, or another vehicle in your flight, you're going to come to a grinding, crumpling, mangling collision with concrete.

"Your skin will be abraded away in spots, loaded with sand, rubber, dust, and bits of dirty gravel in other places. If you land on your head or if, as many cyclists do, you strike your head on the hard surface, you don't have much chance of survival—and perhaps it's just as well, because severe brain damage can ruin your life forever."

How safe is motorcycling compared with driving a car? Your chances of being killed on a motorcycle—per mile ridden—are *20 times* greater than the chances of being killed while driving a car. Head injuries are the greatest risk, and many times arms and legs are broken.

Only the cyclist's skill will protect him from injury, since the vehicle offers no protection. How can you tell skillful from unskillful riders? Here are some of the ways.

SAFE	UNSAFE
Smooth shifting, starting, and stopping	Rapid starts and fast stops
Turning the wheel for slow turns; leaning for higher speed turns	Leaning for slow turns; turning the wheel for higher speed turns
Lower speed on slippery pavements	High speed regardless of conditions
Approved helmet, goggles or face shield; legs and arms covered	No special clothing or equipment

20

Safety as a Passenger

You may think of passengers as being at the mercy of the vehicle operator—and indeed they are. But there are some important passenger skills that help keep the passenger and even the vehicle safe. Maybe you've never considered them before.

Passenger in a Car

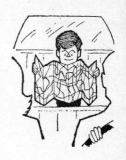

- Don't talk to the driver in a difficult traffic situation. He needs to concentrate on his driving. Don't insist that the radio be on, either.
- Do talk to the driver when he's tired or bored. It will help keep him alert.
- Urge the driver to stop every couple of hours. Bring a ball along and play catch with him in a roadside park if you can. He needs to stretch and get his circulation going.
- Learn to read road maps. You can take strain off the driver by directing him properly and telling him well ahead of turns.
- Use your seat belt. Make sure others use theirs.
- Keep younger children quiet and settle any quarreling fast.
- Lock the doors and see that hands, heads, and feet are kept inside the car—even when parked.

Passenger in a Bus or Train

- Use the handrail to keep your balance in case the vehicle starts up.
- Wait for a complete stop before getting on or off.
- Cross the street behind the bus or after it leaves and you can look for oncoming traffic; don't walk in front of it unless it is a school bus and the driver motions you across while he waits and traffic is stopped.
- Don't talk to or otherwise disturb the bus driver. (This goes for school buses too!)

As you observe passengers, check to see what rules they follow or violate. You may discover some good rules that aren't listed here. If you do, write them down and discuss them with your counselor.

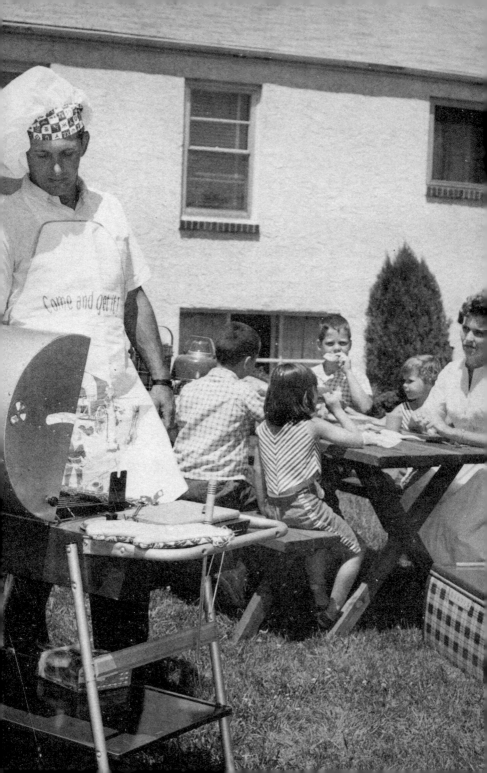

Safety at Home

3. Do the following:

  a. Using a safety checklist approved by your counselor, make an inspection of your home. Explain the hazards found, why they are hazards, and how they can be corrected.

  b. Review your family's plan of escape in case of fire in your home.

Making your home safe does not mean rebuilding it. Neither does it mean purchasing costly new equipment. Safety is simplicity. It may mean disposing of dangerous articles more often than it means acquiring new and safer things. It means refraining from thoughtless and foolhardy actions. It means thinking of safety before you act.

Making your home safe is as easy as keeping house; in fact, the foundation of home safety is good housekeeping. The up-to-date household has a place for everything, and everything is kept in its place. In such a household there is little more that can be done for safety except to make safe practices a matter of daily routine for every member of the family. The checklist offered here has been prepared by the National Safety Council as a guide for good housekeeping and for the prevention of accidents. If you will follow the practices suggested until they become habits in your household, you will be eliminating the major causes of accidental death and injury from your home.

Home Safety Checklists

(Check off each item that describes the situation in your home. If the item is not applicable to your home—for example, if it has to do with stairs and you do not have stairs—skip the item. Each item left represents a hazard or potential hazard.)

Stairways, Halls, and Outside Steps

—— Stairways provided with strong handrail

—— Stairs and halls kept free from boxes, toys, mops, brooms, tools, and other tripping hazards

— Gates at top and bottom of stairs to prevent small children from falling
— Carrying loads so big you can't see where you are going avoided
— Hand free to hold the stair handrail
— Small rugs kept away from the head and foot of stairs
— Stair carpeting or coverings fastened securely
— Stairways and halls have adequate lights, controllable at either end

Kitchen

— Matches put where children cannot get them
— Knives and sharp instruments kept in a special knife drawer or holder out of reach of children
— Can opener used does not leave sharp edges on the can
— Lye, disinfectants, and cleaning products kept out of reach of children
— Pan handles turned away from the stove edges
— Grease, water, or bits of food wiped up immediately if spilled

Bathroom

— Tub and shower equipped with a strong handhold
— Poisons clearly marked (pins in corks or adhesive around bottles to keep containers securely closed)
— All medicines out of reach of children
— Lights turned on before taking medicine

Attic and Basement

— Rubbish and flammable litter kept in covered metal cans pending disposal
— A definite place for children to keep skates, play equipment, etc.
— Walls and beams free from protruding nails
— Electric fuses of the proper size (usually 15 amperes)
— Waste paper kept away from the furnace and the stairs—stacked neatly in bag or box—and clear of possible basement seepage while awaiting disposal

Porch—Yard—Garage

— Railings and banisters sound and inspected periodically
— Steps and walks kept free from ice and snow
— Yard and play space free from holes, stones, broken glass, nail-studded boards, tools, and other litter

— Tools, insecticides, and other dangerous articles out of reach of children
— Wires and low fences brightly painted or marked with cloth strips to make them clearly visible
— Wells, cisterns, and pits kept securely covered
— Children kept away from brush and leaf fires
— Area marked off in garage for bicycles, wagons, etc.

Living Room and Dining Room

— Furniture placed to allow free passage and checked for orderliness at night before retiring
— Furniture and woodwork solid, in good repair, and free from splinters or rough spots
— Fireplace screen fits snugly
— Rugs fastened or laid on a nonslip pad
— Wax on floors thoroughly buffed
— Children taught not to give marbles, jacks, or small toys to baby brothers or sisters
— Fire extinguished in the fireplace before retiring
— Rugs kept from curling at the edges

Bedroom

— Furniture placed to allow clear passage between bed and door and to avoid collision in the dark
— Light switch or lamp located within easy reach from bed
— Bar across bunk beds to prevent falls
— Low-silled windows sturdily screened to prevent children from falling out
— Night lamp in the bedroom and hall for the safety of elderly members of the family
— Smoking in bed prohibited
— Gas and electric heating devices turned off before retiring
— Children taught not to lean against windows or window screens
— Bureau and dressing drawers closed when not in use

Nursery

— Bars on the baby's crib closely spaced so he cannot slip between them
— Baby's crib free from sharp edges or corners
— Sleeping garments and covers that keep the baby warm without danger of smothering or strangling
— Pillows kept out of baby's bassinet or crib
— Thin plastic material not used to cover pillows or mattress

— No toys or objects small enough for baby to swallow or ones that have small components such as eyes that can be removed

— Sturdy toys that do not readily come apart and have no sharp edges or points

— Nonpoisonous paint used when painting baby's furniture and toys

Stoves—Furnaces—Heaters

(These hazards should be checked in all rooms where stoves, furnaces, or other heating devices are used.)

— Stoves located away from windows to avoid setting fire to curtains

— Stove and furnace pipes and flues inspected and cleaned regularly

— Gas burners adjusted properly and free from leaks

— Hot water heater and all small gas or oil room heaters equipped with vent pipes or flues to carry gases of combustion outside of the house

— Flames of gas burners protected from drafts and woodwork within 18 inches of furnace, stove, or heaters protected by an insulating shield

— Nonflammable cleaners provided for use on stoves

— Burnable materials kept well away from heating devices

— Rule against using kerosine to start fires

— Window open for ventilation

Electrical Devices and Fixtures

(These hazards should be checked in all rooms where electrical appliances are used or where electric fixtures are located.)

— All appliances properly grounded electrically

— Electrical fixtures and appliances located and used beyond arm's length of the sink, stove, tub, shower, or other grounded metal objects

— Avoiding touching electrical fixtures or appliances when your hands are wet or when you are standing on a wet floor

— Electric appliances disconnected when only used once in awhile

— Insulating link in the chain on all pull-type sockets

— Household appliance disconnected before attempting to make repairs or adjustments

— Unused, open, screw-type sockets plugged closed.

— Frayed and worn electric cords promptly replaced

— Long, trailing extension cords not in evidence

___ Cords kept out from under rugs, doors, and movable furniture

___ Extension cords of approved type and wire size, used only for temporary hookups

___ Children taught never to touch electric sockets or fixtures

General

(The following hazards should be checked in all parts of your home.)

___ A place for everything and everything in its place

___ Strong rigid stepladder kept in good repair and stored out of the way

___ Window screens and storm windows fastened securely

___ Only nonflammable, low-toxicity dry cleaners used and only outdoors

___ Guns unloaded and stored in locked cases immediately after use (guns and ammunition stored separately)

___ Children given only blunt-end scissors for cutting paper or cloth

___ Clothing free from drooping sleeves, sashes, or frills while doing housework

___ Low-heeled shoes for housework and all shoes in good repair

___ Needles, marbles, and other small or sharp objects kept away from young children

___ Kerosine and gasoline stored in special, clearly marked metal containers outside of the house

___ Metal containers for storage of oil mops, dust rags, painting equipment, and other oily materials.

___ Light turned on before entering a room that is dark

___ Matches out before throwing away

For Emergency

___ Do you know the location of water, gas, and electric shut-off and do you check their operations at least once each year?

___ Do you have a first-aid kit approved by your doctor or the American National Red Cross? Do you keep the supplies replenished?

___ Do you know elementary first-aid procedure?

___ Do you know which is the quickest exit from your home in case of fire?

— Do you know the location of the nearest fire alarm box or how to telephone the fire department?

— Do you know of emergency sources of water existing in your home, if the prime supply should fail? (Water heater, toilet tank, etc.)

— Do you have at hand, for both night and day use, emergency hand lights that can be used on a moment's notice?

— Do you know how to get emergency aid for a member of your family suddenly striken with some attack or illness or injured in some accident?

If so, you're trying to truly "BE PREPARED."

Your Family Escape Plan

Fires in homes are deadly. They often happen at night when occupants are delayed from a prompt escape by sleep. The way to avoid injury or death in a home fire is to get away.

Escaping from a fire in the home sounds easy and sometimes it is. But often people are trapped inside. Many persons are untouched by flames but are asphyxiated (choked) by smoke or gases. There is more to escape from than just flames. A fire that never goes above the basement can kill everyone on the second floor because hot air and smoke rise.

The only way to be reasonably sure of escaping a fire is to have a plan. Then, in case the fire prevents the use of all parts of your plan, you need an alternate escape plan.

Here is the recommendation of the National Safety Council for a family escape plan. Naturally, every family needs to develop its own plan because every house and every family is a little different. But here are the rules from which you can develop your own family escape plan.

• Bedroom doors should be kept *closed* at night. They will delay the spread of a fire and also keep out deadly smoke and gases. The few minutes delay provided by doors may give people the time needed to escape.

• Draw a floor plan of your home. Lay out an escape route for each room on each floor. Then choose an alternate route for each room. (In a fire, the planned escape route might be blocked.) The bedrooms need special attention, because fires at night are usually the most serious.

Escape Tips

- Keep calm.
- Know alternate exit.
- Close door on fire.
- DO NOT REENTER.

DOWNSTAIRS

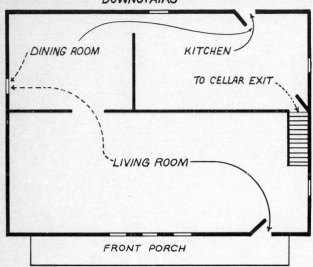

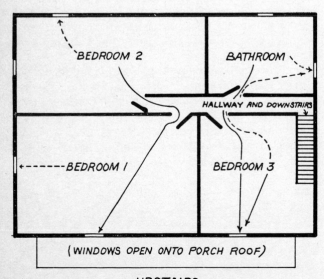

UPSTAIRS

MAIN ROUTE ———→ ALTERNATE ROUTE --------→

Figure 6

Figure 6 on page 29 is a sample escape plan. You can see it as a model for your own.

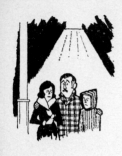

• Very young children and disabled and elderly people will need help in any escape plan. You must include that help in your plan.

• You need a way for every member of the family to awaken the others. You have no way of knowing who might discover a fire while others are sleeping. You can't count on being able to reach all bedrooms; some may be blocked. Yelling, pounding on walls, blowing whistles, etc., may arouse others.

• Teach everyone to escape without wasting time. Getting dressed or gathering valuables can use up precious time.

• Teach everyone how to test a door. If it or the knob is warm, leave it closed and use another route.

• If you must stay in a room, close the door and stay near a slightly opened window. Stuff door cracks with towels or clothing. In a room filled with smoke, crawl with your head about 1½ feet off the floor.

• Decide on a meeting place outside. Thus, you will know when everyone has escaped. (Rescuers are sometimes burned or killed going after someone who has already escaped.)

• Call the fire department only after everyone is out unless someone is trapped inside. Use the nearest phone or alarm box. On the phone, speak clearly and give your name and address. Don't hang up until the other person does.

• When you have set up your escape plan, hold a practice drill. Repeat it from time to time, making changes to allow for a new brother or sister, different sleeping arrangements, etc.

Some Cautions About Your Escape Plan

• Beware of windows that are high, painted shut, or blocked by an air conditioner. They make poor escape routes.

• Make sure escape windows *can* be opened—including screens and storm windows.

• Teach everyone how to break a window with a chair or other heavy object and clear away remaining pieces of glass with a shoe.

• Second-story windows need an emergency ladder, rope, or other escape means unless they open onto some area of refuge like a roof or deck. Bedding can be used in an emergency to help an escape or cushion a fall.

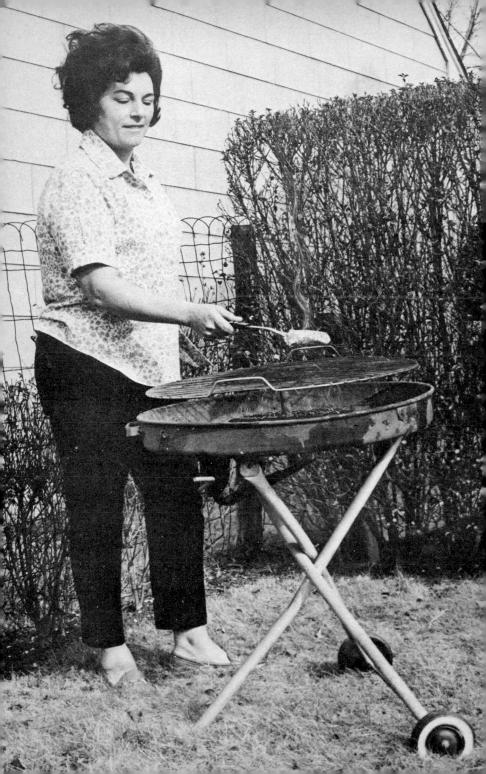

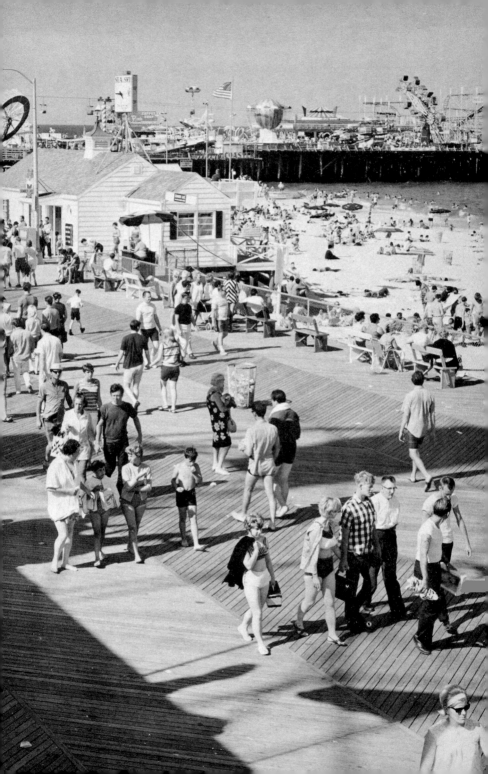

Safety in Public Places

4. Sketch your troop meeting place (or another public building where people gather) and show exits. Are they adequate? Show which exit you would use in an emergency. Explain what should be done in a panic.

Public buildings are often safer than private buildings; that is, they are often built of more fire-resistant materials and have fire exits, emergency lights, doors that open outward, etc.

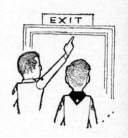

Public places are made hazardous by the people in them. And the hazard created by the people is *panic*.

Panic may or may not be dangerous in a private place. A homeowner may panic in his burning house and run screaming out the door. But he gets out, and no harm is done. Another may panic and "freeze" and later be found dead, although escape would have been easy.

Panic in a public place is deadly. Imagine yourself in a crowded movie theater. Suddenly there is a loud cry: "Fire!" Everyone in the audience rises and runs and pushes toward the front doors. Some fall and are trampled. Bodies pile up in front of the doors, blocking them. Still people push from behind. Perhaps a hundred people die—and there may not be any fire! In a Boston night club, more than 400 people died when fire and panic swept through.

All this means two things to you:

1. You ought to know how to keep yourself from panic.
2. You ought to know how to prevent others from causing panic.

Both of these depend on what you *know*.

Panic and You

Make this a habit: When you attend any public gathering, note the exits before you do anything else. Ask yourself, "If there's trouble here, how can I get out? How can I help other people get out?" Then pick more than one route, just like at home.

Controlling Panic in Others

Most people at a public gathering will not do what you do—note the exits and make a plan to escape. In an emergency, they will rise up and head for the door they entered. It will not occur to most of them that there are other ways out.

What can you do?

1) Just by being calm, you will help. Knowing what to do, you won't panic. That fact alone will help quiet others.

2) Assume calm leadership. Give people around you quiet, firm directions to do something constructive. They will accept them and settle down.

3) Try to turn on lights or otherwise attract attention *to* something *away from* the emergency.

4) Help remove—forcibly if necessary—individuals who have panicked. One screaming person can panic a thousand others.

Where Might You Encounter Emergency in a Public Place?

Emergencies such as fire can happen anywhere. But you are most likely to meet an emergency in public places where you spend the most time.

The 180 or so days you spend in school each year probably make that the most likely public place for you to encounter an emergency. Other likely places: church or synagogue, Scout or Explorer meeting place, theater, library.

Your sketch of your troop or post meeting place will give you good experience in checking public places for exits. Then be sure to use what you know wherever you go.

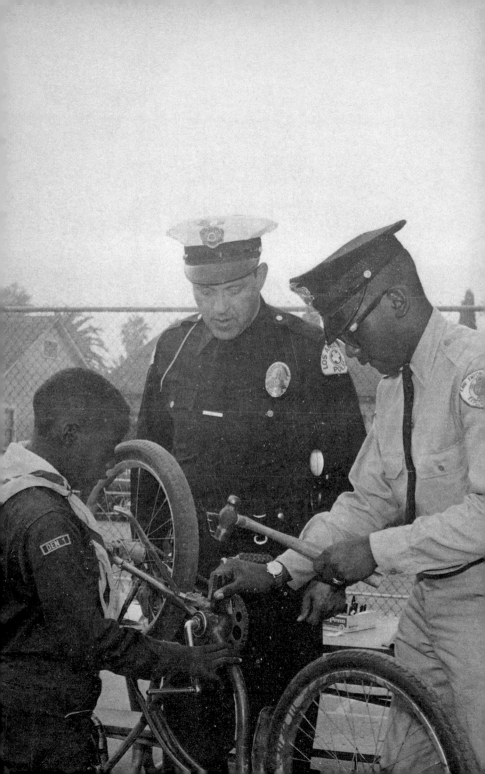

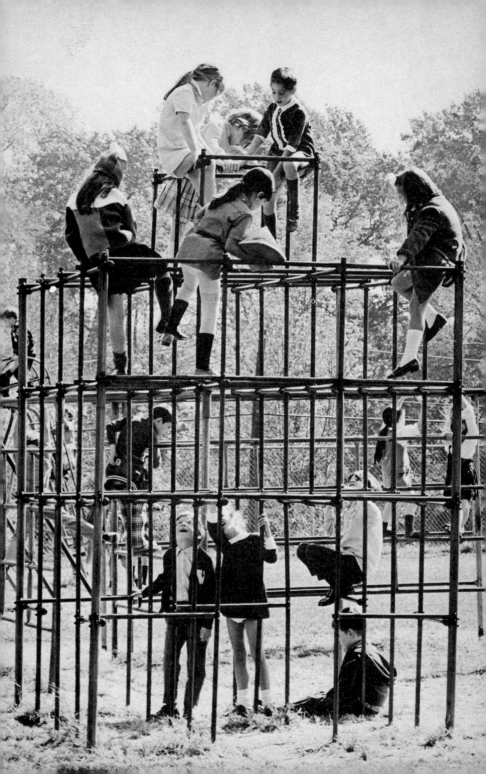

Safety at School and Play

5. Make two safety checklists, one each for school and recreation. Include 10 points on each.

A checklist, remember, can contain both unsafe *conditions* and unsafe *practices*. It will help you to keep them separate while you are making up your lists.

Make the checklists from your own experience and knowledge. You will not learn anything from copying items from existing lists.

In School

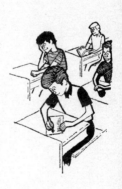

You need not limit your list to practices of students. The building itself and the rules and practices of the school administrators are also part of school safety.

Here are possible types of hazards to check:
- Fire hazard conditions within the building
- Practices that might cause a fire or hinder escape
- Conditions and practices in physical education: gyms, showers, etc.
- Conditions and practices in shops and laboratories
- Backstage conditions and practices in the auditorium
- Waste collection, storage, and disposal

In Recreation

There is no point in making a safety checklist for recreation in general because there is too much to cover. Instead, choose forms of recreation that you enjoy and know about. Don't include reading or watching TV, since such activities don't offer much in the way of hazards.

Sports will offer many opportunities to find and note unsafe practices and conditions. The more exciting a sport is, the more likely it is to have hazards.

Sports and recreation requiring equipment will be more likely to contain hazards in conditions than those that require little equipment. An exception is swimming —a favorite sport of boys your age—requiring no equipment but full of possible unsafe conditions.

The checklist requirement says "at least 10 points." Prove to yourself and your counselor that you really mean business by making it well over the minimum.

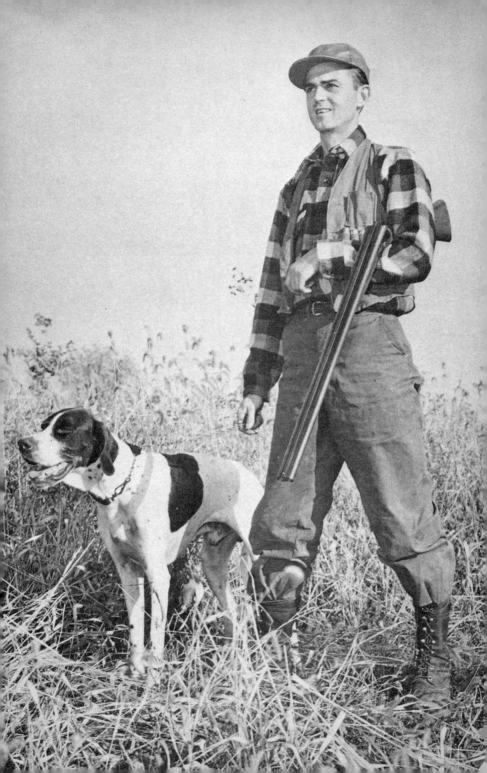

Safety in the Outdoors

6. Make a plan for an accident prevention program for the following outdoor situations: (a) camping and hiking, (b) storm and wind, (c) water activities. Each plan should include an analysis of possible hazards, proposed action to correct the hazards, and reasons for the correction you propose.

Safety becomes more than just an idea when it becomes a *program*. An accident prevention program looks ahead, expects certain types of accidents, and sets out to prevent them. If it's successful, the program actually does prevent many accidents. It also makes accidents that do happen less severe. Let's take a quick look at what has come to be a national accident prevention program.

Many drivers and passengers are hurt or killed when vehicles collide. Studies show that many can escape injury if they could keep from hitting parts of the car: roof, windshield, dashboard, steering wheel. The hazard is the soft, breakable human body being thrown forward into hard, unyielding parts of the car. Such study of accident injuries is called *hazard analysis*.

This analysis shows an unsafe condition. Regardless of what the driver or passengers do or don't do, if there's a collision, they would be thrown into parts of the car—or thrown outside, which is even worse.

The unsafe condition had to be corrected. There had to be action. There are two approaches to this problem. Do you know them?

The first approach was to soften the things the occupants would hit in a collision. This led to such things as collapsible steering columns, padded dashes and visors, and plastic steering wheels that fold up under impact.

The second approach was to hold the occupants in their seats. This started with lap belts and went on to shoulder straps and harnesses.

This accident prevention program is still underway. Many cars are still not properly equipped, and many drivers and passengers still fail to use belts and other safety equipment. But it is a good program, and it contains the same elements that your program will need: analysis of hazards and action.

If you could develop your program in chart form, it would look like this:

CHART OF ACCIDENT PREVENTION PROGRAM

Situation	Hazards	Proposed Action	Reason
Camping	(Your list)	(Your solutions)	(Your reason)
Hiking	"	"	"
Storm and wind	"	"	"
Water activities	"	"	"

Your job in this requirement, then, is to "fill in the blanks." You'll have to find the hazards in these situations, find solutions, and explain why these solutions are the right ones. Here's an example of one camping item:

Hazard—Cutting self with ax

Solutions: 1) Use saws more and axes less.

2) Break up small pieces of wood for the fire instead of chopping them.

3) Require instruction in ax work before allowing Scouts to use axes.

Reasons: 1) Saws are better and safer tools for cutting up wood. Axes should be used only for lopping and splitting.

2) Small dry firewood can be broken faster and more safely than it can be chopped.

3) Axes are dangerous and should not be used by those who have not been taught safe methods.

As you can see, one hazard may need more than one solution. Solutions may involve improving *conditions* or *procedures* or *both*. For example, a sharp ax is safer than a dull ax. But *how you use* an ax, whether dull or sharp, also determines whether you cut yourself.

Here is a good general rule to use. If you can overcome a hazard by making a condition safe, you do it that way. If you can't, then you develop safe ways of doing that hazardous thing. Let's look at an example of each.

Swimming can be hazardous. The danger is drowning. Drowning is caused by water. If you take away the water, you remove the hazard, but, of course, you also take away swimming! So you have to leave the water alone and work on finding ways to swim safely. There are, of course, many safe practices for swimming.

Using flame lights in tents is very hazardous. Gasoline and kerosine lamps, and even candles, have been responsible for many tent fires. But this is an easy hazard to eliminate—you use an electric flashlight instead. You need not develop any safe procedures for using flame lights. You just don't use them—nor do you light matches.

In the case of swimming, you leave the unsafe condition untouched and work on safe ways to swim. In the case of lighting the inside of a tent, you eliminate flame lights, use a harmless flashlight, and forget about any flame safety rules.

Most situations are not all condition or all procedure, however. You may have to do something about both. The dangers of the ax made a good example. Part of the solution was to use a safer tool—*where possible*. When the ax *must* be used, the user must know how to use it safely.

To repeat: Your program of accident prevention consists of analyzing the hazards, finding the solutions, and explaining why these solutions are right.

It's possible that you can develop your accident prevention program from only your own knowledge and experience. But chances are you'll need some help. Your counselor is one source of help. Here are some others—and, of course, there are many more that aren't listed here.

- *Scout Handbook* • *Fieldbook*
- Other merit badge pamphlets
    Camping
    Canoeing
    Cooking
    Firemanship
    First Aid
    Lifesaving
    Personal Fitness
    Pioneering
    Rifle and Shotgun
       Shooting
    Rowing
    Small-Boat Sailing
    Swimming
    Water Skiing

FLAMMABILITY WARNING-CAMPING SAFETY RULES

NO TENT MATERIAL IS FIREPROOF, AND IT CAN BURN WHEN EXPOSED TO HEAT OR FIRE. FOLLOW THESE RULES:

- Only flashlights and electric lanterns are permitted in tents. **NO FLAMES IN TENTS** is a rule which must be enforced.
- Liquid-fuel stoves, heaters, lanterns, lighted candles, matches, or other flame sources should **never** be used in or near tents.
- Do not pitch tents near open fire.
- Do not use flammable chemicals near tents: charcoal lighter, spray cans of paint, bug killer, and repellent.
- Be careful when using electricity and lighting in tents.
- Always extinguish cooking and campfires properly.
- Obey all fire laws, ordinances, and regulations.

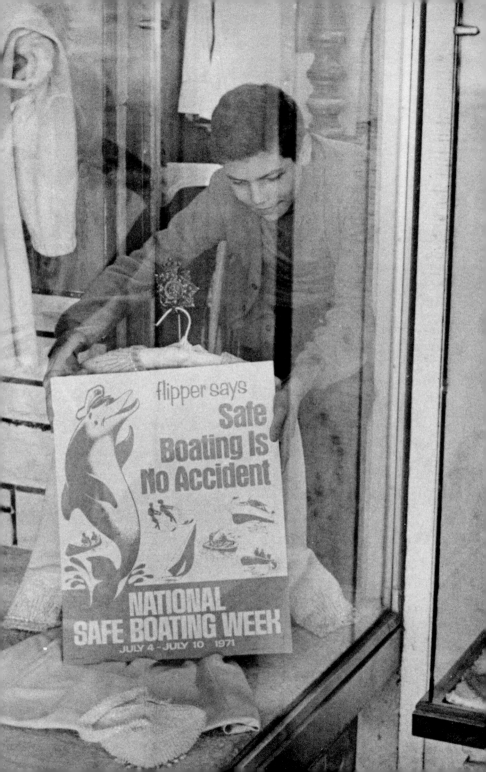

Accident Prevention Projects

7. Do one of the following:

   a. Report on a safety project that you helped to plan or took part in.

   b. Go with a company representative on a safety inspection tour of his company's premises (plant or other place where people work). Make a report.

   c. Join a building or fire inspector on an inspection tour of a public building. Make a report.

   d. Plan a farm safety project to correct unsafe conditions and equipment hazards.

This requirement gives you a chance either to do a safety project or to observe a safety inspection. Which one you choose will depend on what's available to you and what kind of learning experience you want.

Inspection Tours

Going on an inspection tour with a professional safety man can be very helpful. He can show you the checklist he uses, how he spots hidden hazards, how he gets action taken on hazards, and how he trains and motivates people. As a man with a full-time job in safety, he'll be glad to know that you're interested too. One of the best ways to learn about something is to talk with somebody who makes a living at it. Have him tell you how he learned to do what he does. If you want to know about playing the saxophone, then meet a saxophone player. If you want to know about safety, spend some time with a safety professional.

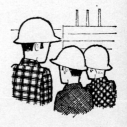

Your Other Choice: A Safety Project

Another good way to learn about something is to do something about it. You'd never learn about swimming if you didn't go near the water.

A project can involve other people. It must be a real project and meet a real need. There's no point in doing a project just to get a badge.

One Scout found that his school library had almost no safety materials. He got some people interested, and some excellent books, pamphlets, and filmstrips were provided.

Another started a bicycle safety program in his town. He got his whole troop involved. Bikes were inspected, instruction was given, and safe-riding contests were held.

Other ideas for community safety projects include:

- Starting a safety poster contest
- Organizing a safety patrol
- Putting on a safety pageant
- Distributing poison-control kits and/or home safety checklist
- Organizing a safety conference
- Making a safety float for a parade
- Operating a safety booth at a fair
- Setting up a safety window display
- Running a drive to eliminate discarded refrigerators with doors or remove doors of abandoned ones.

Remember, these community projects don't have to be done just by you. Safety is more than a one-man job! Other Scouts working on Safety merit badge can help, as can Scout leaders, church and community leaders, service clubs, etc.

If you live on a farm, you'll probably choose the farm safety project. And a farm is a good place to practice safety. The machines and pesticides on farms today have brought a lot of hazards with them.

You can do a real service on the farm by making sure that all machinery has all the proper safety guards and that they all work properly. There are plenty of other kinds of hazards to work on: electric, flooding, lightning, poison, etc. Keeping safe on a farm is no easy job, and you can be a big help.

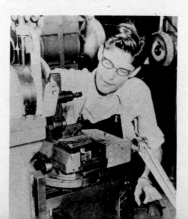

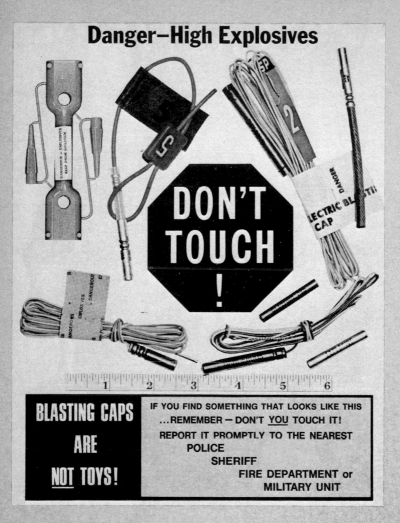

Danger—High Explosives

DON'T TOUCH !

BLASTING CAPS ARE NOT TOYS!

IF YOU FIND SOMETHING THAT LOOKS LIKE THIS
...REMEMBER — DON'T <u>YOU</u> TOUCH IT!
REPORT IT PROMPTLY TO THE NEAREST
POLICE
SHERIFF
FIRE DEPARTMENT or
MILITARY UNIT

Two words tell the basic lesson of blasting cap safety —

DON'T TOUCH!

These small metal tubes —some copper, others aluminum, with or without colored wires, about as big around as a pencil, ¾" to 6 or 7-inches long — are essential tools in construction, mining, quarrying, prospecting and agriculture. They detonate other explosives, and are for use by experts only.

Special care is taken to assure correct use of blasting caps and to provide security in transportation and storage. Occasionally caps are mislaid or stolen. In inexperienced hands they can cause serious injury — or worse.

If you find something that looks like a blasting cap — or the detonating cord connector pictured below — report it promptly to the nearest police or sheriff, fire department or military unit.

This bookmark and related posters are a blasting cap education service of

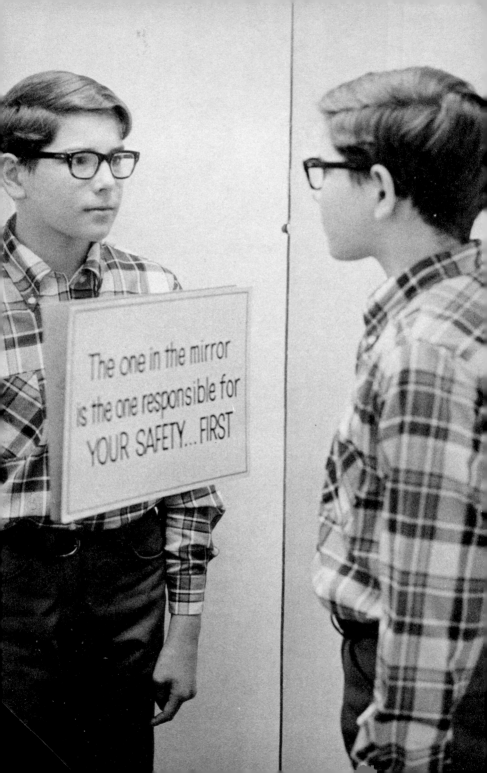

Safety and You

8. Tell how you contribute to the safety of yourself, your family, and your community.

If working on this merit badge does anything for you, it should make you aware of what you do for the safety of yourself and others.

Begin by being honest with yourself about how you keep yourself safe. How much "fooling around" do you do? How many chances do you take to show off? How many times are you doing something dangerous with your mind on something else? And what's going to change now that you've done some study and work in the field of safety?

Are you really helping to keep your family safe? Just what do you do? What have you done? What are you willing to do?

You can't, of course, keep your whole community free of accidents, even if you live in a very small town. But suppose every Scout who earns Safety merit badge did enough to prevent just one serious accident in his community—just one. Thousands of people would be alive and well as a result.

Safety, we hope you have learned, is not something for *sissies*. Talk to any great racing driver, any movie stunt man, any athlete. They'll tell you that safety is a way of life with them. If you're smart, safety will be that way with you, too.

Books About Safety

Recommended by the American Library Association's Advisory Committee to Scouting.

Scout Literature

Archery, Athletics, Automotive Safety, Camping, Canoeing, Cooking, Firemanship, First Aid, Hiking, Horsemanship, Lifesaving, Personal Fitness, Pioneering, Rowing, Rifle and Shotgun Shooting, Skiing, Swimming, and *Water Skiing* merit badge pamphlets
Scout Handbook
Fieldbook

Other Books

The Book of Survival: Everyman's guide to staying alive and handling emergencies in the city, the suburbs, and the wild lands beyond. Anthony Greenback. 1968, Harper.
Coverage of practically every kind of crisis; completely indexed.

The Emergency Book: Jeanne Bendick. 1967, Rand McNally.
How to prevent an emergency as well as how to act during one at home, on the road, with animals, in all sorts of weather, in sports, and in the community.

Fire Prevention: Dorothy Wilson. 1965, F. Watts.
Safety measures to ward off fire, correct procedures where fire is used, what to do in an emergency, and first aid for burns or smoke inhalation.

Basic First Aid: Book 4 of this training series includes water safety and special safety problems. American National Red Cross. 1971, Doubleday.

Motorcycling: Charles Coombs. 1968, Morrow.
Advice on how to select a machine and how to drive; with safety factors stressed throughout.

Stay Alive! Jean Carper. 1965, Doubleday.
Causes of accidents and a guide for protection from fire, poisoning, traffic accidents, drowning, and the dangerous outdoors.

Young People and Driving: The use and abuse of the automobile. Ken W. Purdy. 1967, John Day.
Information about the car, characteristics of good and bad drivers, and tips for safe driving.

The Young Sportsman's Guide to Water Safety: Pat Wilson. 1966, Nelson.
A checklist of safety rules with many instructive photographs.